EASY TYPE 1 DIABETIC VEGETARIAN RECIPES FOR BEGINNERS

Master Plant-Based Cooking for Type 1 Diabetes

By Mia Bennett

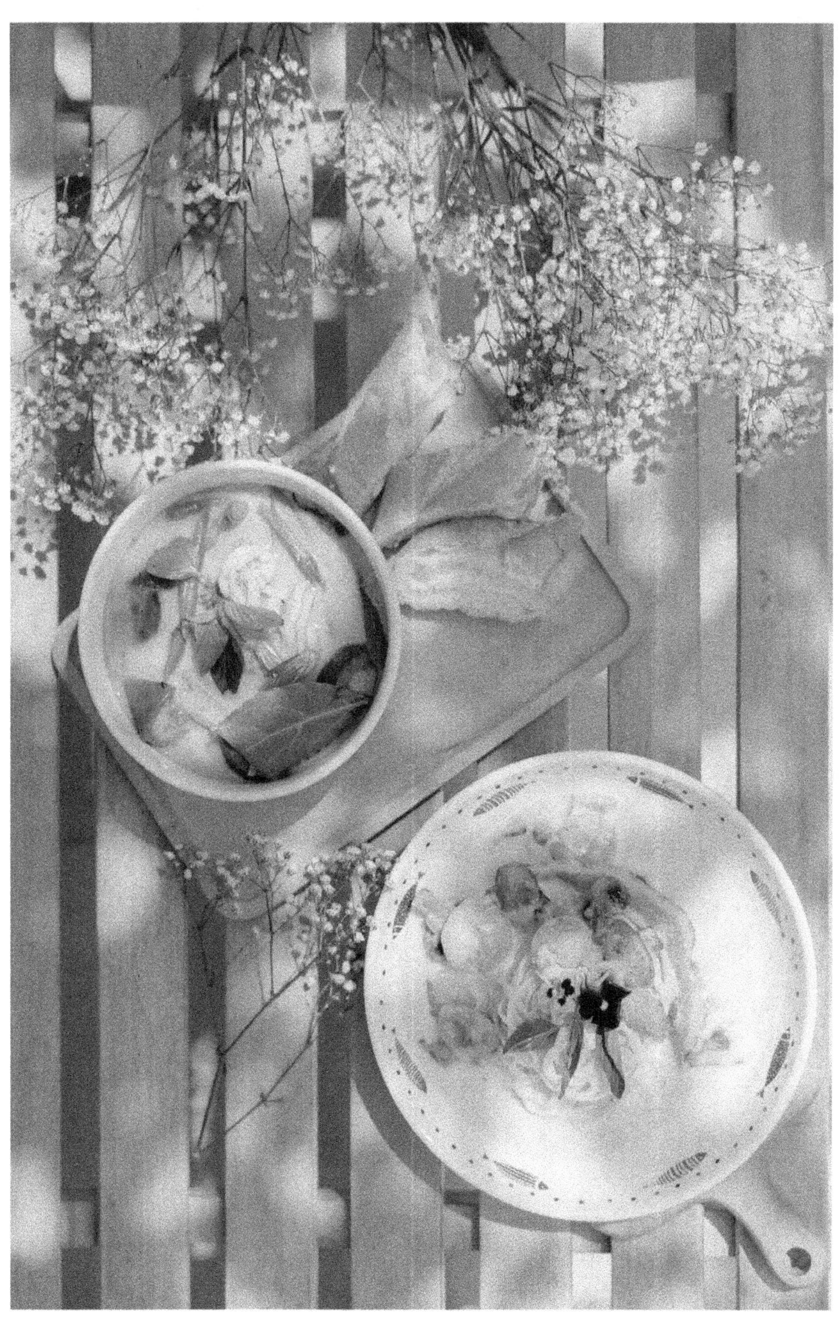

TABLE OF CONTENTS

INTRODUCTION

L iving with type 1 diabetes requires a mindful approach to self-care, and diet plays a crucial role. This guide unpacks the importance of balanced eating, explores the potential benefits of a vegetarian approach, and equips you with tips for meal planning and preparation.

Understanding Type 1 Diabetes:

Unlike type 2 diabetes, where the body produces insulin but struggles to use it effectively, type 1 diabetes is an autoimmune condition. The body's immune system attacks insulin-producing cells, leaving you dependent on injected insulin to manage blood sugar levels. This makes understanding how food impacts your blood sugar (glucose) crucial.

The Power of a Balanced Diet:

A balanced diet is the cornerstone of managing type 1 diabetes. It provides the essential nutrients your body needs while minimizing blood sugar spikes. This typically involves:

- **Non-starchy vegetables**: These are your low-carb friends, packed with vitamins, minerals, and fiber. Think leafy greens, broccoli, peppers, and mushrooms.

- **Whole grains**: Opt for brown rice, quinoa, and whole-wheat bread for sustained energy release.

- **Lean protein sources:** Fish, chicken, beans, and lentils provide essential building blocks and help with satiety.

- **Healthy fats:** Include unsaturated fats from nuts, seeds, and avocado for heart health.

- **Limited fruits**: While fruits offer vitamins, some are high in sugar. Choose berries and apples in moderation.

Exploring Vegetarian Benefits:

While not a magic bullet, research suggests a well-planned vegetarian diet can offer advantages for people with type 1 diabetes:

- **Fiber Powerhouse:** Plant-based meals are naturally high in fiber, which helps regulate blood sugar by slowing down carbohydrate absorption.

- **Weight Management:** Vegetarian diets tend to be lower in calories and fat, promoting weight control, which can improve diabetes management.

- **Heart-Healthy Benefits**: Plant-based fats can lower bad cholesterol (LDL) and improve overall cardiovascular health, a concern for diabetics.

Essential Nutrients and Their Sources:

Here's a quick rundown of key nutrients and where to find them in a vegetarian diet:

- **Protein**: Beans, lentils, tofu, tempeh, nuts, and seeds.
- **Iron**: Dark leafy greens, beans, lentils, fortified cereals, nuts, and seeds.
- **Vitamin B12:** Eggs (for lacto-vegetarians) or fortified foods like cereals and plant-based milk.
- **Calcium**: Dairy products (for lacto-vegetarians) or fortified plant-based milk and leafy greens.

Meal Planning and Preparation Tips:

Conquering mealtimes with type 1 diabetes is all about planning and preparation:

- **Plan your meals:** Dedicate time each week to plan meals and create a grocery list. Consider consulting a registered dietitian for a personalized plan.

- **Stock your pantry:** Keep staples like whole grains, canned beans, nuts, and frozen vegetables on hand for quick and healthy meals.
- **Batch cooking:** Cook large portions on weekends and portion them out for easy weekday meals.
- **Snack smart:** Have healthy grab-and-go options like cut vegetables with hummus or fruits with nut butter.
- **Read food labels:** Pay close attention to carbohydrate content and serving sizes to manage your blood sugar effectively.

Remember: With a balanced approach to food and a supportive healthcare team, you can thrive with type 1 diabetes.

Chapter 2: 30-Day Meal Plan

Week 1

Day 1

- Breakfast: Spinach and Mushroom Omelette
- Lunch: Lentil and Vegetable Soup
- Dinner: Spaghetti Squash with Marinara Sauce
- Snack: Hummus with Veggie Sticks
- Dessert: Chia Seed Pudding with Mango

Day 2

- Breakfast: Greek Yogurt with Berries and Nuts
- Lunch: Quinoa Salad with Chickpeas and Feta
- Dinner: Eggplant Parmesan
- Snack: Roasted Chickpeas
- Dessert: Almond Flour Brownies

Day 3

- Breakfast: Avocado Toast with Cherry Tomatoes
- Lunch: Spinach and Strawberry Salad with Balsamic Vinaigrette
- Dinner: Stuffed Portobello Mushrooms
- Snack: Almond Flour Crackers with Guacamole

- Dessert: Berry Parfait with Greek Yogurt

Day 4

- Breakfast: Oatmeal with Chia Seeds and Blueberries
- Lunch: Veggie Wrap with Hummus
- Dinner: Cauliflower Tacos
- Snack: Greek Yogurt and Cucumber Dip
- Dessert: Coconut Milk Ice Cream

Day 5

- Breakfast: Tofu Scramble with Vegetables
- Lunch: Stuffed Bell Peppers with Brown Rice and Beans
- Dinner: Tofu Stir-Fry with Broccoli and Carrots
- Snack: Edamame with Sea Salt
- Dessert: Baked Apple with Cinnamon and Nuts

Day 6

- Breakfast: Cottage Cheese with Pineapple and Walnuts
- Lunch: Greek Salad with Tofu
- Dinner: Baked Ziti with Spinach
- Snack: Stuffed Mini Bell Peppers
- Dessert: Vegan Chocolate Mousse

Day 7

- Breakfast: Almond Flour Pancakes
- Lunch: Cauliflower Fried Rice
- Dinner: Vegetable Paella
- Snack: Kale Chips
- Dessert: Mixed Berry Crumble

Week 2

Day 8

- Breakfast: Smoothie Bowl with Flaxseeds and Fruits
- Lunch: Black Bean and Corn Salad
- Dinner: Chickpea and Spinach Curry
- Snack: Cottage Cheese and Peach Slices
- Dessert: Avocado Chocolate Pudding

Day 9

- Breakfast: Chia Pudding with Coconut Milk and Strawberries
- Lunch: Roasted Vegetable and Pesto Sandwich
- Dinner: Grilled Vegetable Kebabs
- Snack: Baked Zucchini Fries
- Dessert: Cashew Cheesecake Bites

Day 10

- Breakfast: Whole Wheat Toast with Almond Butter and Sliced Banana
- Lunch: Chickpea and Avocado Salad
- Dinner: Black Bean Enchiladas
- Snack: Avocado Deviled Eggs
- Dessert: Pumpkin Spice Cookies

Day 11

- Breakfast: Vegan Breakfast Burrito
- Lunch: Eggplant and Zucchini Grilled Panini
- Dinner: Sweet Potato and Black Bean Chili
- Snack: Spicy Roasted Almonds
- Dessert: Dark Chocolate and Almond Clusters

Day 12

- Breakfast: Quinoa Porridge with Almonds and Apple Slices
- Lunch: Mixed Greens with Walnuts, Apples, and Blue Cheese
- Dinner: Mushroom and Lentil Shepherd's Pie
- Snack: Tomato and Mozzarella Skewers
- Dessert: Fruit Salad with Mint

Day 13

- Breakfast: Baked Eggplant and Tomato Frittata
- Lunch: Butternut Squash Soup
- Dinner: Zucchini Noodles with Pesto
- Snack: Apple Slices with Peanut Butter
- Dessert: Vegan Lemon Bars

Day 14

- Breakfast: Zucchini and Carrot Muffins
- Lunch: Vegan Sushi Rolls
- Dinner: Vegan Lasagna
- Snack: Carrot and Ginger Soup Shooters
- Dessert: Pear and Almond Tart

Week 3

Day 15

- Breakfast: Cinnamon-Spiced Overnight Oats
- Lunch: Roasted Beet and Goat Cheese Salad
- Dinner: Quinoa-Stuffed Acorn Squash
- Snack: Vegan Stuffed Grape Leaves
- Dessert: Frozen Yogurt Bark with Berries

Day 16

- Breakfast: Spinach and Mushroom Omelette
- Lunch: Lentil and Vegetable Soup
- Dinner: Spaghetti Squash with Marinara Sauce
- Snack: Hummus with Veggie Sticks
- Dessert: Chia Seed Pudding with Mango

Day 17

- Breakfast: Greek Yogurt with Berries and Nuts
- Lunch: Quinoa Salad with Chickpeas and Feta
- Dinner: Eggplant Parmesan
- Snack: Roasted Chickpeas
- Dessert: Almond Flour Brownies

Day 18

- Breakfast: Avocado Toast with Cherry Tomatoes
- Lunch: Spinach and Strawberry Salad with Balsamic Vinaigrette
- Dinner: Stuffed Portobello Mushrooms
- Snack: Almond Flour Crackers with Guacamole
- Dessert: Berry Parfait with Greek Yogurt

Day 19

- Breakfast: Oatmeal with Chia Seeds and Blueberries

- Lunch: Veggie Wrap with Hummus
- Dinner: Cauliflower Tacos
- Snack: Greek Yogurt and Cucumber Dip
- Dessert: Coconut Milk Ice Cream

Day 20

- Breakfast: Tofu Scramble with Vegetables
- Lunch: Stuffed Bell Peppers with Brown Rice and Beans
- Dinner: Tofu Stir-Fry with Broccoli and Carrots
- Snack: Edamame with Sea Salt
- Dessert: Baked Apple with Cinnamon and Nuts

Day 21

- Breakfast: Cottage Cheese with Pineapple and Walnuts
- Lunch: Greek Salad with Tofu
- Dinner: Baked Ziti with Spinach
- Snack: Stuffed Mini Bell Peppers
- Dessert: Vegan Chocolate Mousse

Week 4

Day 22

- Breakfast: Almond Flour Pancakes
- Lunch: Cauliflower Fried Rice

- Dinner: Vegetable Paella
- Snack: Kale Chips
- Dessert: Mixed Berry Crumble

Day 23

- Breakfast: Smoothie Bowl with Flaxseeds and Fruits
- Lunch: Black Bean and Corn Salad
- Dinner: Chickpea and Spinach Curry
- Snack: Cottage Cheese and Peach Slices
- Dessert: Avocado Chocolate Pudding

Day 24

- Breakfast: Chia Pudding with Coconut Milk and Strawberries
- Lunch: Roasted Vegetable and Pesto Sandwich
- Dinner: Grilled Vegetable Kebabs
- Snack: Baked Zucchini Fries
- Dessert: Cashew Cheesecake Bites

Day 25

- Breakfast: Whole Wheat Toast with Almond Butter and Sliced Banana
- Lunch: Chickpea and Avocado Salad
- Dinner: Black Bean Enchiladas

- Snack: Avocado Deviled Eggs
- Dessert: Pumpkin Spice Cookies

Day 26

- Breakfast: Vegan Breakfast Burrito
- Lunch: Eggplant and Zucchini Grilled Panini
- Dinner: Sweet Potato and Black Bean Chili
- Snack: Spicy Roasted Almonds
- Dessert: Dark Chocolate and Almond Clusters

Day 27

- Breakfast: Quinoa Porridge with Almonds and Apple Slices
- Lunch: Mixed Greens with Walnuts, Apples, and Blue Cheese
- Dinner: Mushroom and Lentil Shepherd's Pie
- Snack: Tomato and Mozzarella Skewers
- Dessert: Fruit Salad with Mint

Day 28

- Breakfast: Baked Eggplant and Tomato Frittata
- Lunch: Butternut Squash Soup
- Dinner: Zucchini Noodles with Pesto
- Snack: Apple Slices with Peanut Butter
- Dessert: Vegan Lemon Bars

Day 29

- Breakfast: Zucchini and Carrot Muffins
- Lunch: Vegan Sushi Rolls
- Dinner: Vegan Lasagna
- Snack: Carrot and Ginger Soup Shooters
- Dessert: Pear and Almond Tart

Day 30

- Breakfast: Cinnamon-Spiced Overnight Oats
- Lunch: Roasted Beet and Goat Cheese Salad
- Dinner: Quinoa-Stuffed Acorn Squash
- Snack: Vegan Stuffed Grape Leaves
- Dessert: Frozen Yogurt Bark with Berries

Chapter 2: Breakfast Recipes

Starting your day with a nutritious breakfast is crucial for managing Type 1 diabetes and maintaining energy levels. A balanced breakfast can help stabilize blood sugar levels and keep you satisfied throughout the morning. The following recipes are designed to be simple, delicious, and packed with essential nutrients.

Spinach and Mushroom Omelette

Ingredients:

- 2 eggs
- 1/2 cup spinach, chopped
- 1/4 cup mushrooms, sliced
- 1/4 cup onion, diced
- 1 tbsp olive oil
- Salt and pepper to taste

Instructions:

1. Heat olive oil in a pan over medium heat.
2. Sauté onions and mushrooms until soft.
3. Add spinach and cook until wilted.
4. Beat the eggs in a bowl and season with salt and pepper.

5. Pour eggs into the pan and cook until set, folding the omelette in half.

Nutrition Information (per serving):

- Calories: 210
- Protein: 14g
- Carbohydrates: 5g
- Fat: 16g
- Fiber: 2g
- Sugar: 2g
- Portion Size: 1 omelette

Greek Yogurt with Berries and Nuts

Ingredients:

- 1 cup Greek yogurt
- 1/2 cup mixed berries
- 2 tbsp chopped nuts (almonds, walnuts)
- 1 tsp honey (optional)

Instructions:

1. Spoon Greek yogurt into a bowl.
2. Top with mixed berries and chopped nuts.
3. Drizzle with honey if desired.

Nutrition Information (per serving):

- Calories: 220
- Protein: 15g
- Carbohydrates: 20g
- Fat: 10g
- Fiber: 4g
- Sugar: 12g
- Portion Size: 1 bowl

Avocado Toast with Cherry Tomatoes

Ingredients:

- 1 slice whole grain bread
- 1/2 avocado, mashed
- 5 cherry tomatoes, halved
- Salt and pepper to taste
- Red pepper flakes (optional)

Instructions:

1. Toast the bread slice.
2. Spread mashed avocado on the toast.
3. Top with cherry tomatoes, salt, pepper, and red pepper flakes if using.

Nutrition Information (per serving):

- Calories: 180
- Protein: 4g
- Carbohydrates: 20g
- Fat: 12g
- Fiber: 6g
- Sugar: 3g
- Portion Size: 1 toast

Oatmeal with Chia Seeds and Blueberries

Ingredients:

- 1/2 cup rolled oats
- 1 cup almond milk
- 1 tbsp chia seeds
- 1/2 cup blueberries
- 1 tsp honey (optional)

Instructions:

1. Combine oats, almond milk, and chia seeds in a pot.
2. Cook over medium heat until oats are soft.
3. Stir in blueberries and honey.

Nutrition Information (per serving):

- Calories: 250
- Protein: 6g
- Carbohydrates: 40g
- Fat: 7g
- Fiber: 8g
- Sugar: 10g
- Portion Size: 1 bowl

Tofu Scramble with Vegetables

Ingredients:

- 1/2 block firm tofu, crumbled
- 1/4 cup bell peppers, diced
- 1/4 cup spinach, chopped
- 1/4 cup onions, diced
- 1 tbsp olive oil
- 1/2 tsp turmeric
- Salt and pepper to taste

Instructions:

1. Heat olive oil in a pan over medium heat.
2. Sauté onions and bell peppers until soft.

3. Add crumbled tofu, turmeric, salt, and pepper. Cook until tofu is heated through.

4. Stir in spinach and cook until wilted.

Nutrition Information (per serving):

- Calories: 180
- Protein: 12g
- Carbohydrates: 8g
- Fat: 12g
- Fiber: 4g
- Sugar: 3g
- Portion Size: 1 scramble

Cottage Cheese with Pineapple and Walnuts

Ingredients:

- 1 cup cottage cheese
- 1/2 cup pineapple chunks
- 2 tbsp chopped walnuts

Instructions:

1. Scoop cottage cheese into a bowl.

2. Top with pineapple chunks and chopped walnuts.

Nutrition Information (per serving):

- Calories: 220
- Protein: 18g
- Carbohydrates: 15g
- Fat: 10g
- Fiber: 2g
- Sugar: 10g
- Portion Size: 1 bowl

Almond Flour Pancakes

Ingredients:

- 1 cup almond flour
- 2 eggs
- 1/4 cup almond milk
- 1 tsp baking powder
- 1 tsp vanilla extract
- 1 tbsp coconut oil

Instructions:

1. Mix almond flour, eggs, almond milk, baking powder, and vanilla extract in a bowl.
2. Heat coconut oil in a pan over medium heat.

3. Pour batter into the pan to form pancakes and cook until golden brown on both sides.

Nutrition Information (per serving):

- Calories: 300
- Protein: 12g
- Carbohydrates: 10g
- Fat: 25g
- Fiber: 5g
- Sugar: 2g
- Portion Size: 3 pancakes

Smoothie Bowl with Flaxseeds and Fruits

Ingredients:

- 1 cup frozen mixed berries
- 1 banana
- 1/2 cup almond milk
- 1 tbsp flaxseeds
- Fresh fruit and granola for topping

Instructions:

1. Blend mixed berries, banana, and almond milk until smooth.

2. Pour into a bowl and top with flaxseeds, fresh fruit, and granola.

Nutrition Information (per serving):

- Calories: 250
- Protein: 5g
- Carbohydrates: 50g
- Fat: 6g
- Fiber: 10g
- Sugar: 25g
- Portion Size: 1 bowl

Chia Pudding with Coconut Milk and Strawberries

Ingredients:

- 1/4 cup chia seeds
- 1 cup coconut milk
- 1 tbsp maple syrup
- 1/2 cup strawberries, sliced

Instructions:

1. Mix chia seeds, coconut milk, and maple syrup in a bowl.
2. Refrigerate overnight.

3. Top with sliced strawberries before serving.

Nutrition Information (per serving):

- Calories: 300
- Protein: 5g
- Carbohydrates: 25g
- Fat: 20g
- Fiber: 10g
- Sugar: 10g
- Portion Size: 1 bowl

Whole Wheat Toast with Almond Butter and Sliced Banana

Ingredients:

- 1 slice whole wheat bread
- 1 tbsp almond butter
- 1/2 banana, sliced

Instructions:

1. Toast the bread slice.
2. Spread almond butter on the toast.
3. Top with sliced banana.

Nutrition Information (per serving):

- Calories: 210

- Protein: 6g

- Carbohydrates: 30g

- Fat: 10g

- Fiber: 5g

- Sugar: 10g

- Portion Size: 1 toast

Vegan Breakfast Burrito

Ingredients:

- 1 whole wheat tortilla

- 1/2 cup black beans

- 1/4 cup bell peppers, diced

- 1/4 cup spinach, chopped

- 1/4 avocado, sliced

- Salsa to taste

Instructions:

1. Warm the tortilla in a pan.

2. Fill with black beans, bell peppers, spinach, and avocado.

3. Add salsa and roll up the tortilla.

Nutrition Information (per serving):

- Calories: 300
- Protein: 10g
- Carbohydrates: 45g
- Fat: 10g
- Fiber: 12g
- Sugar: 2g
- Portion Size: 1 burrito

Quinoa Porridge with Almonds and Apple Slices

Ingredients:

- 1/2 cup quinoa
- 1 cup almond milk
- 1 tbsp maple syrup
- 1/2 apple, sliced
- 2 tbsp chopped almonds

Instructions:

1. Cook quinoa in almond milk until soft.
2. Stir in maple syrup.
3. Top with apple slices and chopped almonds.

Nutrition Information (per serving):

- Calories: 250
- Protein: 8g
- Carbohydrates: 40g
- Fat: 8g
- Fiber: 6g
- Sugar: 15g
- Portion Size: 1 bowl

Baked Eggplant and Tomato Frittata

Ingredients:

- 1/2 eggplant, sliced
- 1 cup cherry tomatoes, halved
- 4 eggs
- 1/4 cup milk
- 1 tbsp olive oil
- Salt and pepper to taste

Instructions:

1. Preheat oven to 375°F (190°C).
2. Sauté eggplant slices in olive oil until soft.
3. Arrange eggplant and cherry tomatoes in a baking dish.

4. Beat eggs with milk, salt, and pepper, then pour over vegetables.

5. Bake for 20 minutes or until set.

Nutrition Information (per serving):

- Calories: 200
- Protein: 12g
- Carbohydrates: 10g
- Fat: 14g
- Fiber: 4g
- Sugar: 6g
- Portion Size: 1 slice

Zucchini and Carrot Muffins

Ingredients:

- 1 cup grated zucchini
- 1 cup grated carrot
- 2 eggs
- 1 cup almond flour
- 1/4 cup coconut oil, melted
- 1 tsp baking soda
- 1 tsp cinnamon

Instructions:

1. Preheat oven to 350°F (175°C).
2. Mix zucchini, carrot, eggs, almond flour, coconut oil, baking soda, and cinnamon in a bowl.
3. Pour batter into muffin tins.
4. Bake for 25 minutes or until a toothpick comes out clean.

Nutrition Information (per serving):

- Calories: 150
- Protein: 5g
- Carbohydrates: 10g
- Fat: 10g
- Fiber: 3g
- Sugar: 5g
- Portion Size: 1 muffin

Cinnamon-Spiced Overnight Oats

Ingredients:

- 1/2 cup rolled oats
- 1/2 cup almond milk
- 1/2 tsp cinnamon
- 1 tbsp chia seeds
- 1 tbsp maple syrup

Instructions:

1. Combine oats, almond milk, cinnamon, chia seeds, and maple syrup in a jar.
2. Refrigerate overnight.
3. Stir before serving.

Nutrition Information (per serving):

- Calories: 200
- Protein: 6g
- Carbohydrates: 35g
- Fat: 5g
- Fiber: 7g
- Sugar: 10g
- Portion Size: 1 jar

Chapter 3: Lunch Recipes

A well-balanced lunch is crucial for maintaining stable blood sugar levels and sustaining energy throughout the day, especially for those managing Type 1 diabetes. These vegetarian lunch recipes are designed to be nutritious, delicious, and easy to prepare.

Lentil and Vegetable Soup

Ingredients:

- 1 cup lentils, rinsed
- 1 onion, diced
- 2 carrots, sliced
- 2 celery stalks, sliced
- 3 cloves garlic, minced
- 1 zucchini, diced
- 1 can (14.5 oz) diced tomatoes
- 6 cups vegetable broth
- 1 tsp thyme
- Salt and pepper to taste

Instructions:

1. In a large pot, sauté onion, carrots, celery, and garlic until softened.

2. Add lentils, tomatoes, and broth. Bring to a boil.

3. Reduce heat and simmer for 30 minutes.

4. Add zucchini and thyme. Cook for another 10 minutes.

5. Season with salt and pepper.

Nutrition Information (per serving):

- Calories: 220
- Protein: 12g
- Carbohydrates: 38g
- Fat: 2g
- Fiber: 12g
- Sugar: 8g
- Portion size: 1 bowl

Quinoa Salad with Chickpeas and Feta

Ingredients:

- 1 cup quinoa, cooked
- 1 can (15 oz) chickpeas, drained and rinsed
- 1 cup cherry tomatoes, halved
- 1 cucumber, diced
- 1/2 red onion, diced
- 1/2 cup feta cheese, crumbled
- 2 tbsp olive oil

- 1 tbsp lemon juice

- Salt and pepper to taste

Instructions:

1. In a large bowl, combine quinoa, chickpeas, tomatoes, cucumber, and red onion.

2. Drizzle with olive oil and lemon juice.

3. Toss to combine.

4. Top with crumbled feta cheese.

5. Season with salt and pepper.

Nutrition Information (per serving):

- Calories: 320

- Protein: 12g

- Carbohydrates: 42g

- Fat: 12g

- Fiber: 8g

- Sugar: 6g

- Portion size: 1 cup

Spinach and Strawberry Salad with Balsamic Vinaigrette

Ingredients:

- 4 cups baby spinach
- 1 cup strawberries, sliced
- 1/4 cup walnuts, chopped
- 1/4 cup crumbled goat cheese
- 2 tbsp balsamic vinegar
- 1 tbsp olive oil
- Salt and pepper to taste

Instructions:

1. In a large bowl, combine spinach, strawberries, walnuts, and goat cheese.
2. In a small bowl, whisk together balsamic vinegar and olive oil.
3. Drizzle vinaigrette over the salad.
4. Toss gently to combine.
5. Season with salt and pepper.

Nutrition Information (per serving):

- Calories: 210
- Protein: 6g
- Carbohydrates: 14g

- Fat: 15g

- Fiber: 4g

- Sugar: 8g

- Portion size: 1 cup

Veggie Wrap with Hummus

Ingredients:

- 1 whole wheat tortilla

- 1/2 cup hummus

- 1/2 cup shredded carrots

- 1/2 cup sliced cucumbers

- 1/2 cup bell peppers, sliced

- 1/4 cup red cabbage, shredded

- 1/4 cup baby spinach

Instructions:

1. Spread hummus evenly over the tortilla.

2. Layer with carrots, cucumbers, bell peppers, red cabbage, and spinach.

3. Roll up the tortilla tightly.

4. Cut in half and serve.

Nutrition Information (per serving):

- Calories: 300
- Protein: 8g
- Carbohydrates: 42g
- Fat: 10g
- Fiber: 8g
- Sugar: 6g
- Portion size: 1 wrap

Stuffed Bell Peppers with Brown Rice and Beans

Ingredients:

- 4 bell peppers, tops cut off and seeds removed
- 1 cup cooked brown rice
- 1 can (15 oz) black beans, drained and rinsed
- 1 cup corn kernels
- 1 cup diced tomatoes
- 1 tsp cumin
- Salt and pepper to taste

Instructions:

1. Preheat oven to 375°F (190°C).

2. In a bowl, mix brown rice, black beans, corn, tomatoes, and cumin.

3. Stuff the bell peppers with the mixture.

4. Place stuffed peppers in a baking dish.

5. Cover with foil and bake for 30 minutes.

6. Remove foil and bake for another 10 minutes.

Nutrition Information (per serving):

- Calories: 280
- Protein: 10g
- Carbohydrates: 52g
- Fat: 2g
- Fiber: 10g
- Sugar: 8g
- Portion size: 1 stuffed pepper

Greek Salad with Tofu

Ingredients:

- 1 block firm tofu, cubed
- 1 cucumber, diced
- 1 cup cherry tomatoes, halved
- 1/2 red onion, sliced
- 1/4 cup Kalamata olives, pitted

- 1/4 cup feta cheese, crumbled
- 2 tbsp olive oil
- 1 tbsp red wine vinegar
- 1 tsp dried oregano
- Salt and pepper to taste

Instructions:

1. In a bowl, combine tofu, cucumber, tomatoes, red onion, and olives.
2. Drizzle with olive oil and red wine vinegar.
3. Sprinkle with oregano.
4. Toss gently to combine.
5. Top with crumbled feta cheese.
6. Season with salt and pepper.

Nutrition Information (per serving):

- Calories: 270
- Protein: 14g
- Carbohydrates: 16g
- Fat: 18g
- Fiber: 4g
- Sugar: 6g
- Portion size: 1 cup

Cauliflower Fried Rice

Ingredients:

- 1 head cauliflower, grated
- 1 cup frozen peas and carrots
- 1 small onion, diced
- 2 cloves garlic, minced
- 2 eggs, beaten
- 2 tbsp soy sauce
- 1 tbsp sesame oil
- 2 green onions, sliced

Instructions:

1. Heat sesame oil in a large skillet over medium heat.
2. Add onion and garlic, cook until fragrant.
3. Add grated cauliflower and cook for 5 minutes.
4. Stir in peas and carrots, cook for another 3 minutes.
5. Push mixture to the side, scramble eggs in the skillet.
6. Mix scrambled eggs into the cauliflower.
7. Stir in soy sauce and green onions.

Nutrition Information (per serving):

- Calories: 200
- Protein: 10g
- Carbohydrates: 16g

- Fat: 12g
- Fiber: 6g
- Sugar: 4g
- Portion size: 1 cup

Black Bean and Corn Salad

Ingredients:

- 1 can (15 oz) black beans, drained and rinsed
- 1 cup corn kernels
- 1 red bell pepper, diced
- 1/4 red onion, diced
- 1/4 cup cilantro, chopped
- 2 tbsp lime juice
- 1 tbsp olive oil
- Salt and pepper to taste

Instructions:

1. In a bowl, combine black beans, corn, bell pepper, red onion, and cilantro.
2. Drizzle with lime juice and olive oil.
3. Toss to combine.
4. Season with salt and pepper.

Nutrition Information (per serving):

- Calories: 180
- Protein: 8g
- Carbohydrates: 30g
- Fat: 4g
- Fiber: 10g
- Sugar: 4g
- Portion size: 1 cup

Roasted Vegetable and Pesto Sandwich

Ingredients:

- 1 zucchini, sliced
- 1 red bell pepper, sliced
- 1 yellow bell pepper, sliced
- 1 eggplant, sliced
- 2 tbsp olive oil
- Salt and pepper to taste
- 4 slices whole grain bread
- 1/4 cup pesto

Instructions:

1. Preheat oven to 400°F (200°C).

2. Toss zucchini, bell peppers, and eggplant with olive oil, salt, and pepper.

3. Roast vegetables on a baking sheet for 20 minutes.

4. Spread pesto on one side of each bread slice.

5. Layer roasted vegetables on two slices of bread.

6. Top with the remaining bread slices, pesto side down.

7. Grill sandwiches in a pan until golden brown.

Nutrition Information (per serving):

- Calories: 320
- Protein: 8g
- Carbohydrates: 40g
- Fat: 14g
- Fiber: 8g
- Sugar: 6g
- Portion size: 1 sandwich

Chickpea and Avocado Salad

Ingredients:

- 1 can (15 oz) chickpeas, drained and rinsed
- 1 avocado, diced
- 1/2 red onion, diced
- 1/4 cup cilantro, chopped

- 2 tbsp lime juice

- 1 tbsp olive oil

- Salt and pepper to taste

Instructions:

1. In a bowl, combine chickpeas, avocado, red onion, and cilantro.
2. Drizzle with lime juice and olive oil.
3. Toss gently to combine.
4. Season with salt and pepper.

Nutrition Information (per serving):

- Calories: 250
- Protein: 8g
- Carbohydrates: 28g
- Fat: 14g
- Fiber: 10g
- Sugar: 3g
- Portion size: 1 cup

Eggplant and Zucchini Grilled Panini

Ingredients:

- 1 small eggplant, sliced

- 1 zucchini, sliced
- 4 slices whole grain bread
- 2 tbsp olive oil
- 1/4 cup goat cheese
- Salt and pepper to taste

Instructions:

1. Preheat a grill pan over medium heat.
2. Brush eggplant and zucchini slices with olive oil, season with salt and pepper.
3. Grill vegetables until tender and grill marks appear.
4. Spread goat cheese on one side of each bread slice.
5. Layer grilled vegetables on two slices of bread.
6. Top with remaining bread slices, goat cheese side down.
7. Grill sandwiches until golden brown.

Nutrition Information (per serving):

- Calories: 340
- Protein: 10g
- Carbohydrates: 44g
- Fat: 16g
- Fiber: 8g
- Sugar: 6g
- Portion size: 1 panini

Mixed Greens with Walnuts, Apples, and Blue Cheese

Ingredients:

- 4 cups mixed greens
- 1 apple, sliced
- 1/4 cup walnuts, chopped
- 1/4 cup crumbled blue cheese
- 2 tbsp balsamic vinaigrette

Instructions:

1. In a large bowl, combine mixed greens, apple slices, and walnuts.
2. Top with crumbled blue cheese.
3. Drizzle with balsamic vinaigrette.
4. Toss gently to combine.

Nutrition Information (per serving):

- Calories: 230
- Protein: 6g
- Carbohydrates: 18g
- Fat: 16g
- Fiber: 4g
- Sugar: 12g
- Portion size: 1 cup

Butternut Squash Soup

Ingredients:

- 1 butternut squash, peeled and cubed
- 1 onion, diced
- 2 cloves garlic, minced
- 4 cups vegetable broth
- 1/2 tsp nutmeg
- Salt and pepper to taste

Instructions:

1. In a large pot, sauté onion and garlic until softened.
2. Add butternut squash and vegetable broth. Bring to a boil.
3. Reduce heat and simmer until squash is tender.
4. Puree the soup using an immersion blender.
5. Stir in nutmeg, salt, and pepper.

Nutrition Information (per serving):

- Calories: 180
- Protein: 4g
- Carbohydrates: 38g
- Fat: 1g
- Fiber: 7g
- Sugar: 8g
- Portion size: 1 bowl

Vegan Sushi Rolls

Ingredients:

- 1 cup sushi rice, cooked
- 4 nori sheets
- 1 avocado, sliced
- 1 cucumber, julienned
- 1 carrot, julienned
- Soy sauce for serving

Instructions:

1. Lay nori sheet on a bamboo mat.
2. Spread a thin layer of sushi rice over nori.
3. Arrange avocado, cucumber, and carrot strips along one edge.
4. Roll nori tightly using the bamboo mat.
5. Slice into bite-sized pieces.
6. Serve with soy sauce.

Nutrition Information (per serving):

- Calories: 220
- Protein: 4g
- Carbohydrates: 40g
- Fat: 6g
- Fiber: 5g

- Sugar: 2g
- Portion size: 1 roll

Roasted Beet and Goat Cheese Salad

Ingredients:

- 4 cups mixed greens
- 2 beets, roasted and sliced
- 1/4 cup goat cheese, crumbled
- 1/4 cup walnuts, chopped
- 2 tbsp balsamic vinaigrette

Instructions:

1. In a large bowl, combine mixed greens and roasted beets.
2. Top with crumbled goat cheese and walnuts.
3. Drizzle with balsamic vinaigrette.
4. Toss gently to combine.

Nutrition Information (per serving):

- Calories: 240
- Protein: 6g
- Carbohydrates: 20g
- Fat: 16g
- Fiber: 5g

- Sugar: 10g
- Portion size: 1 cup

Chapter 4: Dinner Recipes

Dinner is an essential meal of the day, providing a chance to unwind and refuel after a busy day. For those with Type 1 diabetes, choosing the right dinner recipes can help maintain blood sugar levels while also enjoying delicious, satisfying meals. This chapter presents easy-to-make vegetarian dinner recipes, each packed with nutrients and tailored for beginners.

Spaghetti Squash with Marinara Sauce

Ingredients:

- 1 large spaghetti squash
- 2 cups marinara sauce
- 1 tablespoon olive oil
- Salt and pepper to taste
- Fresh basil for garnish

Instructions:

1. Preheat oven to 400°F (200°C). Cut the spaghetti squash in half lengthwise and remove seeds.
2. Drizzle with olive oil, salt, and pepper. Place cut side down on a baking sheet and bake for 40 minutes.

3. Remove squash from oven and use a fork to scrape out the "spaghetti" strands.

4. Heat marinara sauce in a saucepan. Serve the spaghetti squash topped with marinara and fresh basil.

Nutrition Information:

- Calories: 120
- Protein: 2g
- Carbohydrates: 20g
- Fat: 4g
- Fiber: 4g
- Sugar: 8g
- Portion Size: 1 cup

Eggplant Parmesan

Ingredients:

- 1 large eggplant, sliced
- 2 cups marinara sauce
- 1 cup shredded mozzarella cheese
- 1 cup grated Parmesan cheese
- 1 cup breadcrumbs
- 1 tablespoon olive oil

Instructions:

1. Preheat oven to 375°F (190°C). Sprinkle eggplant slices with salt and let sit for 30 minutes. Pat dry.
2. Dip each slice in olive oil, then breadcrumbs.
3. Arrange on a baking sheet and bake for 20 minutes, flipping halfway.
4. Layer a baking dish with marinara sauce, eggplant slices, mozzarella, and Parmesan. Repeat layers.
5. Bake for 25 minutes until cheese is melted and bubbly.

Nutrition Information:

*   Calories: 250
*   Protein: 12g
*   Carbohydrates: 28g
*   Fat: 12g
*   Fiber: 8g
*   Sugar: 10g
*   Portion Size: 1 slice

Stuffed Portobello Mushrooms

Ingredients:

*   4 large Portobello mushrooms
*   1 cup spinach, chopped

- 1 cup ricotta cheese
- 1/4 cup grated Parmesan cheese
- 1 clove garlic, minced
- Salt and pepper to taste

Instructions:

1. Preheat oven to 375°F (190°C). Remove stems from mushrooms and scoop out gills.
2. Mix spinach, ricotta, Parmesan, garlic, salt, and pepper in a bowl.
3. Stuff mushrooms with the mixture and place on a baking sheet.
4. Bake for 20 minutes until mushrooms are tender.

Nutrition Information:

- Calories: 180
- Protein: 12g
- Carbohydrates: 8g
- Fat: 12g
- Fiber: 3g
- Sugar: 2g
- Portion Size: 1 mushroom

Cauliflower Tacos

Ingredients:

- 1 head cauliflower, cut into florets
- 1 tablespoon olive oil
- 1 teaspoon cumin
- 1 teaspoon chili powder
- Salt and pepper to taste
- 8 small corn tortillas
- 1 cup shredded cabbage
- 1 avocado, sliced
- Salsa and lime wedges for serving

Instructions:

1. Preheat oven to 400°F (200°C). Toss cauliflower with olive oil, cumin, chili powder, salt, and pepper.
2. Spread on a baking sheet and roast for 25 minutes until golden.
3. Warm tortillas and fill with roasted cauliflower, cabbage, and avocado.
4. Serve with salsa and lime wedges.

Nutrition Information:

- Calories: 220
- Protein: 4g

- Carbohydrates: 28g

- Fat: 10g

- Fiber: 8g

- Sugar: 3g

- Portion Size: 2 tacos

Tofu Stir-Fry with Broccoli and Carrots

Ingredients:

- 1 block firm tofu, cubed

- 2 cups broccoli florets

- 2 carrots, sliced

- 1 tablespoon soy sauce

- 1 tablespoon sesame oil

- 1 clove garlic, minced

- 1 tablespoon grated ginger

Instructions:

1. Heat sesame oil in a large skillet over medium heat. Add tofu and cook until golden.

2. Add garlic and ginger, sauté for 1 minute.

3. Add broccoli and carrots, stir-fry for 5 minutes.

4. Stir in soy sauce and cook for another 2 minutes.

Nutrition Information:

- Calories: 210
- Protein: 12g
- Carbohydrates: 12g
- Fat: 14g
- Fiber: 4g
- Sugar: 4g
- Portion Size: 1 cup

Baked Ziti with Spinach

Ingredients:

- 8 oz whole wheat ziti pasta
- 2 cups marinara sauce
- 1 cup ricotta cheese
- 1 cup shredded mozzarella cheese
- 2 cups spinach, chopped
- 1 tablespoon olive oil

Instructions:

1. Preheat oven to 375°F (190°C). Cook pasta according to package instructions.
2. Mix cooked pasta with marinara sauce, ricotta, spinach, and half the mozzarella.

3. Transfer to a baking dish and top with remaining mozzarella.

4. Bake for 20 minutes until cheese is melted and bubbly.

Nutrition Information:

- Calories: 300
- Protein: 15g
- Carbohydrates: 42g
- Fat: 10g
- Fiber: 6g
- Sugar: 8g
- Portion Size: 1 cup

Vegetable Paella

Ingredients:

- 1 cup Arborio rice
- 1 bell pepper, diced
- 1 zucchini, diced
- 1 cup green beans, trimmed
- 1 cup peas
- 1 onion, chopped
- 3 cloves garlic, minced
- 1 teaspoon smoked paprika
- 1/4 teaspoon saffron threads

- 4 cups vegetable broth

Instructions:

1. Heat olive oil in a large pan over medium heat. Sauté onion and garlic until soft.
2. Add bell pepper, zucchini, green beans, and peas. Cook for 5 minutes.
3. Stir in rice, smoked paprika, and saffron.
4. Add vegetable broth, bring to a boil, then simmer for 20 minutes until rice is tender.

Nutrition Information:

- Calories: 250
- Protein: 6g
- Carbohydrates: 45g
- Fat: 5g
- Fiber: 5g
- Sugar: 6g
- Portion Size: 1 cup

Chickpea and Spinach Curry

Ingredients:

- 1 can chickpeas, drained and rinsed

- 2 cups spinach, chopped
- 1 onion, chopped
- 2 cloves garlic, minced
- 1 tablespoon curry powder
- 1 can coconut milk
- 1 tablespoon olive oil

Instructions:

1. Heat olive oil in a large pot over medium heat. Sauté onion and garlic until golden.
2. Add curry powder and cook for 1 minute.
3. Stir in chickpeas, spinach, and coconut milk. Simmer for 10 minutes until spinach is wilted.

Nutrition Information:

- Calories: 280
- Protein: 8g
- Carbohydrates: 28g
- Fat: 16g
- Fiber: 6g
- Sugar: 4g
- Portion Size: 1 cup

Grilled Vegetable Kebabs

Ingredients:

- 1 zucchini, sliced
- 1 bell pepper, cut into squares
- 1 red onion, cut into squares
- 1 cup cherry tomatoes
- 1/4 cup olive oil
- 2 tablespoons balsamic vinegar
- Salt and pepper to taste

Instructions:

1. Preheat grill to medium-high heat. Thread vegetables onto skewers.
2. Mix olive oil, balsamic vinegar, salt, and pepper. Brush over vegetables.
3. Grill for 10-15 minutes, turning occasionally, until vegetables are tender.

Nutrition Information:

- Calories: 150
- Protein: 2g
- Carbohydrates: 12g
- Fat: 12g
- Fiber: 3g

- Sugar: 6g
- Portion Size: 2 kebabs

Black Bean Enchiladas

Ingredients:

- 1 can black beans, drained and rinsed
- 8 small corn tortillas
- 1 cup enchilada sauce
- 1 cup shredded cheese
- 1 cup corn kernels
- 1 tablespoon olive oil

Instructions:

1. Preheat oven to 375°F (190°C). Mix black beans and corn in a bowl.
2. Warm tortillas and fill with bean mixture. Roll and place in a baking dish.
3. Pour enchilada sauce over tortillas and sprinkle with cheese.
4. Bake for 20 minutes until cheese is melted and bubbly.

Nutrition Information:

- Calories: 300
- Protein: 12g

- Carbohydrates: 40g

- Fat: 10g

- Fiber: 10g

- Sugar: 6g

- Portion Size: 2 enchiladas

Sweet Potato and Black Bean Chili

Ingredients:

- 2 sweet potatoes, diced

- 1 can black beans, drained and rinsed

- 1 onion, chopped

- 2 cloves garlic, minced

- 1 can diced tomatoes

- 2 cups vegetable broth

- 1 tablespoon chili powder

- 1 teaspoon cumin

- Salt and pepper to taste

Instructions:

1. Heat olive oil in a large pot over medium heat. Sauté onion and garlic until golden.

2. Add sweet potatoes, black beans, tomatoes, broth, chili powder, and cumin.

3. Bring to a boil, then simmer for 30 minutes until sweet potatoes are tender.

Nutrition Information:

- Calories: 280
- Protein: 10g
- Carbohydrates: 52g
- Fat: 4g
- Fiber: 14g
- Sugar: 8g
- Portion Size: 1 cup

Mushroom and Lentil Shepherd's Pie

Ingredients:

- 1 cup lentils, cooked
- 2 cups mushrooms, sliced
- 1 onion, chopped
- 2 carrots, diced
- 2 cloves garlic, minced
- 1 cup vegetable broth
- 1 tablespoon tomato paste
- 4 cups mashed potatoes

Instructions:

1. Preheat oven to 375°F (190°C). Sauté onion, garlic, carrots, and mushrooms in a large pan until tender.

2. Add lentils, broth, and tomato paste. Cook for 10 minutes.

3. Transfer mixture to a baking dish and spread mashed potatoes on top.

4. Bake for 20 minutes until top is golden.

Nutrition Information:

- Calories: 350
- Protein: 14g
- Carbohydrates: 60g
- Fat: 6g
- Fiber: 12g
- Sugar: 6g
- Portion Size: 1 cup

Zucchini Noodles with Pesto

Ingredients:

- 4 zucchinis, spiralized
- 1 cup fresh basil leaves
- 1/4 cup pine nuts
- 1/4 cup Parmesan cheese

- 1/4 cup olive oil

- 2 cloves garlic, minced

- Salt and pepper to taste

Instructions:

1. Blend basil, pine nuts, Parmesan, olive oil, garlic, salt, and pepper to make pesto.

2. Toss zucchini noodles with pesto.

3. Serve immediately or sauté for 2 minutes for a warm dish.

Nutrition Information:

- Calories: 200

- Protein: 6g

- Carbohydrates: 8g

- Fat: 18g

- Fiber: 3g

- Sugar: 5g

- Portion Size: 1 cup

Vegan Lasagna

Ingredients:

- 12 lasagna noodles

- 3 cups marinara sauce

- 1 cup vegan ricotta cheese
- 2 cups spinach, chopped
- 1 cup sliced mushrooms
- 1 tablespoon olive oil

Instructions:

1. Preheat oven to 375°F (190°C). Cook lasagna noodles according to package instructions.
2. Layer a baking dish with marinara, noodles, ricotta, spinach, and mushrooms. Repeat layers.
3. Bake for 30 minutes until bubbly and golden.

Nutrition Information:

- Calories: 350
- Protein: 12g
- Carbohydrates: 50g
- Fat: 10g
- Fiber: 8g
- Sugar: 12g
- Portion Size: 1 slice

Quinoa-Stuffed Acorn Squash

Ingredients:

- 2 acorn squashes, halved and seeded
- 1 cup quinoa, cooked
- 1 apple, diced
- 1/4 cup dried cranberries
- 1/4 cup chopped pecans
- 1 tablespoon olive oil
- 1 teaspoon cinnamon

Instructions:

1. Preheat oven to 400°F (200°C). Brush squash halves with olive oil and sprinkle with cinnamon.
2. Roast squash for 40 minutes until tender.
3. Mix quinoa, apple, cranberries, and pecans.
4. Fill squash halves with quinoa mixture and serve.

Nutrition Information:

- Calories: 300
- Protein: 6g
- Carbohydrates: 52g
- Fat: 10g
- Fiber: 8g
- Sugar: 15g
- Portion Size: 1 half squash

Chapter 5: Snacks and Appetizers

Snacking can be an essential part of a balanced diet, especially for those managing Type 1 diabetes. It's important to choose snacks that provide sustained energy, are rich in nutrients, and help maintain stable blood sugar levels. This chapter offers a variety of easy-to-prepare vegetarian snacks and appetizers that are not only healthy but also delicious.

Hummus with Veggie Sticks

Ingredients:

- 1 can chickpeas, drained and rinsed
- 1/4 cup tahini
- 2 tablespoons olive oil
- 1 clove garlic, minced
- Juice of 1 lemon
- Salt to taste
- Assorted veggie sticks (carrots, cucumbers, bell peppers)

Instructions:

1. In a food processor, combine chickpeas, tahini, olive oil, garlic, lemon juice, and salt.
2. Blend until smooth.

3. Serve with assorted veggie sticks.

Nutrition Information:

- Calories: 200
- Protein: 6g
- Carbohydrates: 16g
- Fat: 12g
- Fiber: 4g
- Sugar: 2g
- Portion Size: 1/4 cup hummus with 1 cup veggie sticks

Roasted Chickpeas

Ingredients:

- 1 can chickpeas, drained and rinsed
- 1 tablespoon olive oil
- 1 teaspoon smoked paprika
- 1/2 teaspoon garlic powder
- Salt to taste

Instructions:

1. Preheat oven to 400°F.
2. Toss chickpeas with olive oil, smoked paprika, garlic powder, and salt.

3. Spread on a baking sheet and roast for 25-30 minutes until crispy.

Nutrition Information:

- Calories: 120
- Protein: 5g
- Carbohydrates: 20g
- Fat: 3g
- Fiber: 6g
- Sugar: 1g
- Portion Size: 1/2 cup

Almond Flour Crackers with Guacamole

Ingredients:

- 1 cup almond flour
- 1 tablespoon flaxseed meal
- 1/4 teaspoon salt
- 1 egg
- 2 ripe avocados
- 1 lime, juiced
- 1/4 cup diced red onion
- Salt and pepper to taste

Instructions:

1. Preheat oven to 350°F.
2. Mix almond flour, flaxseed meal, salt, and egg to form a dough.
3. Roll out dough between parchment paper and cut into crackers.
4. Bake for 10-12 minutes until golden.
5. Mash avocados with lime juice, red onion, salt, and pepper to make guacamole.
6. Serve crackers with guacamole.

Nutrition Information:

- Calories: 250
- Protein: 8g
- Carbohydrates: 10g
- Fat: 20g
- Fiber: 8g
- Sugar: 1g
- Portion Size: 6-8 crackers with 1/4 cup guacamole

Greek Yogurt and Cucumber Dip

Ingredients:

- 1 cup Greek yogurt

- 1/2 cucumber, grated and drained
- 1 clove garlic, minced
- 1 tablespoon chopped fresh dill
- Salt and pepper to taste

Instructions:

1. Combine Greek yogurt, grated cucumber, garlic, dill, salt, and pepper in a bowl.
2. Mix well and chill before serving.

Nutrition Information:

- Calories: 100
- Protein: 10g
- Carbohydrates: 6g
- Fat: 3g
- Fiber: 0g
- Sugar: 4g
- Portion Size: 1/2 cup

Edamame with Sea Salt

Ingredients:

- 1 cup edamame (in pods)
- Sea salt to taste

Instructions:

1. Steam or boil edamame for 5 minutes until tender.

2. Sprinkle with sea salt and serve warm.

Nutrition Information:

- Calories: 120

- Protein: 11g

- Carbohydrates: 10g

- Fat: 5g

- Fiber: 4g

- Sugar: 2g

- Portion Size: 1 cup

Stuffed Mini Bell Peppers

Ingredients:

- 12 mini bell peppers

- 1 cup cooked quinoa

- 1/2 cup black beans, drained and rinsed

- 1/4 cup chopped fresh cilantro

- 1 tablespoon lime juice

- Salt and pepper to taste

Instructions:

1. Cut tops off mini bell peppers and remove seeds.

2. Mix quinoa, black beans, cilantro, lime juice, salt, and pepper in a bowl.

3. Stuff mixture into bell peppers.

Nutrition Information:

- Calories: 150
- Protein: 5g
- Carbohydrates: 25g
- Fat: 2g
- Fiber: 6g
- Sugar: 4g
- Portion Size: 3 stuffed peppers

Kale Chips

Ingredients:

- 1 bunch kale, stems removed and leaves torn
- 1 tablespoon olive oil
- Salt to taste

Instructions:

1. Preheat oven to 350°F.

2. Toss kale leaves with olive oil and salt.

3. Spread on a baking sheet and bake for 10-15 minutes until crispy.

Nutrition Information:

- Calories: 50
- Protein: 2g
- Carbohydrates: 7g
- Fat: 2g
- Fiber: 2g
- Sugar: 0g
- Portion Size: 1 cup

Cottage Cheese and Peach Slices

Ingredients:

- 1 cup cottage cheese
- 1 peach, sliced

Instructions:

1. Spoon cottage cheese into a bowl.
2. Top with peach slices.

Nutrition Information:

- Calories: 150

- Protein: 14g

- Carbohydrates: 12g

- Fat: 5g

- Fiber: 1g

- Sugar: 9g

- Portion Size: 1 cup

Baked Zucchini Fries

Ingredients:

- 2 zucchinis, cut into fries

- 1/2 cup almond flour

- 1/4 cup grated Parmesan cheese

- 1 egg, beaten

- Salt and pepper to taste

Instructions:

1. Preheat oven to 425°F.

2. Mix almond flour, Parmesan, salt, and pepper.

3. Dip zucchini fries in egg, then coat with almond flour mixture.

4. Place on a baking sheet and bake for 20 minutes until crispy.

Nutrition Information:

- Calories: 130
- Protein: 6g
- Carbohydrates: 8g
- Fat: 8g
- Fiber: 3g
- Sugar: 3g
- Portion Size: 1 cup

Avocado Deviled Eggs

Ingredients:

- 6 hard-boiled eggs, halved
- 1 avocado
- 1 tablespoon lime juice
- 1/4 cup diced red onion
- Salt and pepper to taste

Instructions:

1. Scoop yolks from eggs and mix with avocado, lime juice, red onion, salt, and pepper.
2. Spoon mixture back into egg whites.

Nutrition Information:

- Calories: 100
- Protein: 6g
- Carbohydrates: 3g
- Fat: 8g
- Fiber: 2g
- Sugar: 1g
- Portion Size: 2 halves

Spicy Roasted Almonds

Ingredients:

- 1 cup raw almonds
- 1 tablespoon olive oil
- 1 teaspoon chili powder
- 1/2 teaspoon cumin
- Salt to taste

Instructions:

1. Preheat oven to 350°F.
2. Toss almonds with olive oil, chili powder, cumin, and salt.
3. Spread on a baking sheet and roast for 15 minutes.

Nutrition Information:

- Calories: 200
- Protein: 6g
- Carbohydrates: 7g
- Fat: 18g
- Fiber: 4g
- Sugar: 1g
- Portion Size: 1/4 cup

Tomato and Mozzarella Skewers

Ingredients:

- 12 cherry tomatoes
- 12 small mozzarella balls
- Fresh basil leaves
- Balsamic glaze

Instructions:

1. Skewer cherry tomatoes, mozzarella balls, and basil leaves.
2. Drizzle with balsamic glaze before serving.

Nutrition Information:

- Calories: 100
- Protein: 6g

- Carbohydrates: 3g
- Fat: 7g
- Fiber: 1g
- Sugar: 2g
- Portion Size: 4 skewers

Apple Slices with Peanut Butter

Ingredients:

- 1 apple, sliced
- 2 tablespoons peanut butter

Instructions:

1. Slice apple.
2. Serve with peanut butter for dipping.

Nutrition Information:

- Calories: 200
- Protein: 4g
- Carbohydrates: 26g
- Fat: 10g
- Fiber: 4g
- Sugar: 19g
- Portion Size: 1 apple with 2 tablespoons peanut butter

Carrot and Ginger Soup Shooters

Ingredients:

- 4 large carrots, peeled and chopped
- 1 tablespoon olive oil
- 1 onion, chopped
- 1 clove garlic, minced
- 1 teaspoon grated fresh ginger
- 4 cups vegetable broth
- Salt and pepper to taste

Instructions:

1. Sauté carrots, onion, garlic, and ginger in olive oil until tender.
2. Add vegetable broth and simmer for 20 minutes.
3. Blend until smooth and season with salt and pepper.
4. Serve in small shooter glasses.

Nutrition Information:

- Calories: 70
- Protein: 1g
- Carbohydrates: 10g
- Fat: 3g
- Fiber: 2g
- Sugar: 5g

- Portion Size: 1 shooter (4 oz)

Vegan Stuffed Grape Leaves

Ingredients:

- 1 jar grape leaves, rinsed and drained
- 1 cup cooked rice
- 1/4 cup pine nuts
- 1/4 cup currants
- 1 tablespoon chopped fresh dill
- 1 tablespoon lemon juice
- Salt and pepper to taste

Instructions:

1. Mix rice, pine nuts, currants, dill, lemon juice, salt, and pepper.
2. Place a spoonful of mixture on each grape leaf and roll tightly.
3. Chill before serving.

Nutrition Information:

- Calories: 100
- Protein: 2g
- Carbohydrates: 15g

- Fat: 3g
- Fiber: 2g
- Sugar: 1g
- Portion Size: 4 grape leaves

Chapter 6: Desserts

Desserts are often the highlight of any meal, bringing sweetness and satisfaction to the end of your culinary journey. In this chapter, we explore a variety of delectable desserts that cater to diverse dietary preferences and cravings. Whether you're a seasoned baker or a novice in the kitchen, these recipes are designed to be straightforward and rewarding.

Chia Seed Pudding with Mango

Ingredients:

- 1/4 cup chia seeds
- 1 cup almond milk
- 1 tablespoon maple syrup
- 1 teaspoon vanilla extract
- 1 ripe mango, diced

Instructions:

1. Mix chia seeds, almond milk, maple syrup, and vanilla extract in a bowl.
2. Refrigerate for at least 2 hours or overnight until it thickens.
3. Top with diced mango before serving.

Nutrition Information:

- Calories: 200
- Protein: 4g
- Carbohydrates: 30g
- Fat: 9g
- Fiber: 10g
- Sugar: 18g
- Portion Size: 1 cup

Almond Flour Brownies

Ingredients:

- 1 cup almond flour
- 1/2 cup cocoa powder
- 1/2 teaspoon baking powder
- 1/4 teaspoon salt
- 1/2 cup coconut sugar
- 1/3 cup melted coconut oil
- 2 eggs
- 1 teaspoon vanilla extract

Instructions:

1. Preheat oven to 350°F (175°C). Grease a baking pan.

2. Mix almond flour, cocoa powder, baking powder, and salt in a bowl.

3. In another bowl, whisk coconut sugar, coconut oil, eggs, and vanilla extract.

4. Combine wet and dry ingredients. Pour into the baking pan.

5. Bake for 20-25 minutes. Cool before cutting.

Nutrition Information:

- Calories: 210

- Protein: 5g

- Carbohydrates: 15g

- Fat: 15g

- Fiber: 4g

- Sugar: 10g

- Portion Size: 1 brownie

Berry Parfait with Greek Yogurt

Ingredients:

- 1 cup Greek yogurt

- 1/2 cup mixed berries (strawberries, blueberries, raspberries)

- 1 tablespoon honey

- 1/4 cup granola

Instructions:

1. Layer Greek yogurt, berries, honey, and granola in a glass.

2. Repeat layers until all ingredients are used.

3. Serve immediately.

Nutrition Information:

- Calories: 250
- Protein: 12g
- Carbohydrates: 32g
- Fat: 8g
- Fiber: 5g
- Sugar: 20g
- Portion Size: 1 parfait

Coconut Milk Ice Cream

Ingredients:

- 2 cups coconut milk
- 1/2 cup sugar
- 1 teaspoon vanilla extract

Instructions:

1. Mix coconut milk, sugar, and vanilla extract in a bowl.

2. Pour into an ice cream maker and churn according to manufacturer's instructions.

3. Freeze for 2 hours before serving.

Nutrition Information:

- Calories: 240
- Protein: 2g
- Carbohydrates: 25g
- Fat: 15g
- Fiber: 0g
- Sugar: 20g
- Portion Size: 1/2 cup

Baked Apple with Cinnamon and Nuts

Ingredients:

- 2 apples, cored
- 2 tablespoons chopped nuts (walnuts or pecans)
- 1 tablespoon honey
- 1 teaspoon cinnamon

Instructions:

1. Preheat oven to 350°F (175°C).

2. Place cored apples in a baking dish.

3. Fill with nuts, drizzle with honey, and sprinkle with
   cinnamon.

4. Bake for 25-30 minutes until tender.

Nutrition Information:

- Calories: 180
- Protein: 2g
- Carbohydrates: 30g
- Fat: 6g
- Fiber: 5g
- Sugar: 22g
- Portion Size: 1 apple

Vegan Chocolate Mousse

Ingredients:

- 1 ripe avocado
- 1/4 cup cocoa powder
- 1/4 cup maple syrup
- 1 teaspoon vanilla extract
- Pinch of salt

Instructions:

1. Blend avocado, cocoa powder, maple syrup, vanilla extract, and salt until smooth.
2. Chill for 1 hour before serving.

Nutrition Information:

- Calories: 200
- Protein: 3g
- Carbohydrates: 25g
- Fat: 11g
- Fiber: 8g
- Sugar: 18g
- Portion Size: 1/2 cup

Mixed Berry Crumble

Ingredients:

- 2 cups mixed berries (strawberries, blueberries, raspberries)
- 1/4 cup rolled oats
- 1/4 cup almond flour
- 2 tablespoons coconut oil, melted
- 2 tablespoons maple syrup

Instructions:

1. Preheat oven to 350°F (175°C).
2. Place berries in a baking dish.
3. Mix oats, almond flour, coconut oil, and maple syrup in a bowl. Sprinkle over berries.
4. Bake for 20-25 minutes until topping is golden.

Nutrition Information:

- Calories: 180
- Protein: 3g
- Carbohydrates: 28g
- Fat: 8g
- Fiber: 6g
- Sugar: 18g
- Portion Size: 1/2 cup

Avocado Chocolate Pudding

Ingredients:

- 1 ripe avocado
- 1/4 cup cocoa powder
- 1/4 cup honey
- 1/4 cup almond milk
- 1 teaspoon vanilla extract

Instructions:

1. Blend avocado, cocoa powder, honey, almond milk, and vanilla extract until smooth.
2. Chill for 1 hour before serving.

Nutrition Information:

- Calories: 220
- Protein: 3g
- Carbohydrates: 30g
- Fat: 12g
- Fiber: 8g
- Sugar: 22g
- Portion Size: 1/2 cup

Cashew Cheesecake Bites

Ingredients:

- 1 cup raw cashews, soaked overnight
- 1/4 cup coconut oil, melted
- 1/4 cup maple syrup
- 1 teaspoon vanilla extract
- 1 tablespoon lemon juice

Instructions:

1. Blend soaked cashews, coconut oil, maple syrup, vanilla extract, and lemon juice until smooth.
2. Pour into mini muffin tins. Freeze for 2 hours before serving.

Nutrition Information:

*   Calories: 150
*   Protein: 3g
*   Carbohydrates: 10g
*   Fat: 12g
*   Fiber: 1g
*   Sugar: 6g
*   Portion Size: 1 bite

Pumpkin Spice Cookies

Ingredients:

*   1 cup pumpkin puree
*   1/2 cup coconut sugar
*   1/4 cup coconut oil, melted
*   1 teaspoon vanilla extract
*   1 cup almond flour
*   1/2 teaspoon baking soda
*   1 teaspoon pumpkin spice

Instructions:

1. Preheat oven to 350°F (175°C). Line a baking sheet with parchment paper.
2. Mix pumpkin puree, coconut sugar, coconut oil, and vanilla extract in a bowl.
3. Add almond flour, baking soda, and pumpkin spice. Mix until combined.
4. Drop spoonfuls of dough onto the baking sheet.
5. Bake for 12-15 minutes. Cool before serving.

Nutrition Information:

- Calories: 120
- Protein: 2g
- Carbohydrates: 14g
- Fat: 6g
- Fiber: 2g
- Sugar: 7g
- Portion Size: 1 cookie

Dark Chocolate and Almond Clusters

Ingredients:

- 1 cup dark chocolate chips
- 1/2 cup almonds, chopped

Instructions:

1. Melt dark chocolate chips in a microwave or double boiler.
2. Stir in chopped almonds.
3. Drop spoonfuls onto a parchment-lined baking sheet.
4. Chill until set, about 30 minutes.

Nutrition Information:

- Calories: 150
- Protein: 3g
- Carbohydrates: 12g
- Fat: 11g
- Fiber: 3g
- Sugar: 7g
- Portion Size: 2 clusters

Fruit Salad with Mint

Ingredients:

- 1 cup diced pineapple
- 1 cup diced watermelon
- 1 cup sliced strawberries
- 1 tablespoon chopped fresh mint
- 1 tablespoon lime juice

Instructions:

1. Mix pineapple, watermelon, strawberries, mint, and lime juice in a bowl.
2. Chill for 30 minutes before serving.

Nutrition Information:

- Calories: 70
- Protein: 1g
- Carbohydrates: 18g
- Fat: 0g
- Fiber: 2g
- Sugar: 15g
- Portion Size: 1 cup

Vegan Lemon Bars

Ingredients:

- 1 cup almond flour
- 1/4 cup coconut oil, melted
- 2 tablespoons maple syrup
- 1/2 cup lemon juice
- 1/4 cup coconut sugar
- 2 tablespoons cornstarch

Instructions:

1. Preheat oven to 350°F (175°C). Line a baking pan with parchment paper.
2. Mix almond flour, coconut oil, and maple syrup. Press into the pan.
3. Bake for 10 minutes.
4. Mix lemon juice, coconut sugar, and cornstarch. Pour over crust.
5. Bake for another 20 minutes. Cool before cutting.

Nutrition Information:

- Calories: 140
- Protein: 2g
- Carbohydrates: 15g
- Fat: 9g
- Fiber: 2g
- Sugar: 8g
- Portion Size: 1 bar

Pear and Almond Tart

Ingredients:

- 1 pre-made pie crust
- 2 ripe pears, sliced

- 1/4 cup almond flour

- 2 tablespoons coconut sugar

- 1 tablespoon melted coconut oil

- 1 teaspoon cinnamon

Instructions:

1. Preheat oven to 350°F (175°C).

2. Place pie crust in a tart pan. Arrange pear slices on top.

3. Mix almond flour, coconut sugar, coconut oil, and cinnamon. Sprinkle over pears.

4. Bake for 25-30 minutes until golden.

Nutrition Information:

- Calories: 220

- Protein: 3g

- Carbohydrates: 30g

- Fat: 10g

- Fiber: 4g

- Sugar: 14g

- Portion Size: 1 slice

Frozen Yogurt Bark with Berries

Ingredients:

- 2 cups Greek yogurt
- 1/4 cup honey
- 1 cup mixed berries (strawberries, blueberries, raspberries)

Instructions:

1. Mix Greek yogurt and honey.
2. Spread onto a parchment-lined baking sheet.
3. Sprinkle with mixed berries.
4. Freeze for 2 hours. Break into pieces before serving.

Nutrition Information:

- Calories: 100
- Protein: 5g
- Carbohydrates: 18g
- Fat: 2g
- Fiber: 2g
- Sugar: 14g
- Portion Size: 1 piece

Chapter 7: Smoothies

In this chapter, we'll explore different smoothie recipes, each with its own unique blend of flavors and health benefits. From detoxifying greens to indulgent chocolate blends, there's something for everyone. Each recipe is designed to be simple to follow, requiring only a few ingredients and a blender.

Green Detox Smoothie

Ingredients:

- 1 cup spinach
- 1 green apple, chopped
- 1/2 cucumber
- 1 lemon, juiced
- 1-inch piece of ginger
- 1 cup water

Instructions:

1. Combine all ingredients in a blender.
2. Blend until smooth.
3. Serve immediately.

Nutrition Information (per serving):

- Calories: 90
- Protein: 1g
- Carbohydrates: 22g
- Fat: 0g
- Fiber: 5g
- Sugar: 13g
- Portion Size: 1 cup

Berry and Spinach Smoothie

Ingredients:

- 1 cup mixed berries (strawberries, blueberries, raspberries)
- 1 cup spinach
- 1 banana
- 1 cup almond milk

Instructions:

1. Place all ingredients in a blender.
2. Blend until smooth.
3. Pour into a glass and enjoy.

Nutrition Information (per serving):

- Calories: 150

- Protein: 2g

- Carbohydrates: 34g

- Fat: 2g

- Fiber: 7g

- Sugar: 18g

- Portion Size: 1.5 cups

Mango and Turmeric Smoothie

Ingredients:

- 1 cup frozen mango chunks

- 1/2 teaspoon turmeric powder

- 1/2 cup coconut milk

- 1/2 cup orange juice

Instructions:

1. Add all ingredients to a blender.

2. Blend until smooth.

3. Serve chilled.

Nutrition Information (per serving):

- Calories: 160

- Protein: 1g

- Carbohydrates: 36g

- Fat: 4g
- Fiber: 3g
- Sugar: 28g
- Portion Size: 1 cup

Peanut Butter Banana Smoothie

Ingredients:

- 1 banana
- 2 tablespoons peanut butter
- 1 cup milk (dairy or plant-based)
- 1 tablespoon honey (optional)

Instructions:

1. Place all ingredients in a blender.
2. Blend until smooth and creamy.
3. Pour into a glass and enjoy.

Nutrition Information (per serving):

- Calories: 300
- Protein: 8g
- Carbohydrates: 36g
- Fat: 16g
- Fiber: 4g

- Sugar: 20g
- Portion Size: 1.5 cups

Kale and Pineapple Smoothie

Ingredients:

- 1 cup kale, stems removed
- 1/2 cup pineapple chunks
- 1 banana
- 1 cup coconut water

Instructions:

1. Add all ingredients to a blender.
2. Blend until smooth.
3. Serve immediately.

Nutrition Information (per serving):

- Calories: 120
- Protein: 2g
- Carbohydrates: 30g
- Fat: 0g
- Fiber: 4g
- Sugar: 20g
- Portion Size: 1 cup

Avocado and Berry Smoothie

Ingredients:

- 1/2 avocado
- 1 cup mixed berries
- 1 cup almond milk
- 1 tablespoon honey

Instructions:

1. Combine all ingredients in a blender.
2. Blend until smooth.
3. Serve chilled.

Nutrition Information (per serving):

- Calories: 200
- Protein: 3g
- Carbohydrates: 30g
- Fat: 10g
- Fiber: 8g
- Sugar: 18g
- Portion Size: 1.5 cups

Apple Pie Smoothie

Ingredients:

- 1 apple, chopped
- 1/2 teaspoon cinnamon
- 1/4 teaspoon nutmeg
- 1 cup vanilla yogurt
- 1/2 cup milk

Instructions:

1. Place all ingredients in a blender.
2. Blend until smooth.
3. Pour into a glass and enjoy.

Nutrition Information (per serving):

- Calories: 180
- Protein: 6g
- Carbohydrates: 36g
- Fat: 3g
- Fiber: 4g
- Sugar: 28g
- Portion Size: 1.5 cups

Carrot and Ginger Smoothie

Ingredients:

- 1 cup carrot juice
- 1 banana
- 1/2 teaspoon fresh ginger, grated
- 1/2 cup orange juice

Instructions:

1. Combine all ingredients in a blender.
2. Blend until smooth.
3. Serve immediately.

Nutrition Information (per serving):

- Calories: 130
- Protein: 1g
- Carbohydrates: 32g
- Fat: 0g
- Fiber: 3g
- Sugar: 20g
- Portion Size: 1 cup

Chocolate Protein Smoothie

Ingredients:

- 1 scoop chocolate protein powder
- 1 banana
- 1 tablespoon cocoa powder
- 1 cup milk (dairy or plant-based)

Instructions:

1. Add all ingredients to a blender.
2. Blend until smooth.
3. Serve chilled.

Nutrition Information (per serving):

- Calories: 250
- Protein: 20g
- Carbohydrates: 30g
- Fat: 6g
- Fiber: 5g
- Sugar: 15g
- Portion Size: 1.5 cups

Blueberry and Almond Smoothie

Ingredients:

- 1 cup blueberries
- 1 tablespoon almond butter
- 1 cup almond milk
- 1 teaspoon honey

Instructions:

1. Combine all ingredients in a blender.
2. Blend until smooth.
3. Serve immediately.

Nutrition Information (per serving):

- Calories: 180
- Protein: 4g
- Carbohydrates: 25g
- Fat: 8g
- Fiber: 5g
- Sugar: 15g
- Portion Size: 1 cup

Tropical Green Smoothie

Ingredients:

- 1/2 cup pineapple chunks
- 1/2 cup mango chunks
- 1 cup spinach
- 1 cup coconut water

Instructions:

1. Add all ingredients to a blender.
2. Blend until smooth.
3. Serve chilled.

Nutrition Information (per serving):

- Calories: 140
- Protein: 2g
- Carbohydrates: 35g
- Fat: 0g
- Fiber: 3g
- Sugar: 25g
- Portion Size: 1 cup

Beetroot and Berry Smoothie

Ingredients:

- 1 small beetroot, cooked and chopped
- 1 cup mixed berries
- 1 banana
- 1 cup apple juice

Instructions:

1. Combine all ingredients in a blender.
2. Blend until smooth.
3. Serve immediately.

Nutrition Information (per serving):

- Calories: 160
- Protein: 2g
- Carbohydrates: 38g
- Fat: 0g
- Fiber: 5g
- Sugar: 30g
- Portion Size: 1.5 cups

Coconut and Mango Smoothie

Ingredients:

- 1 cup frozen mango chunks
- 1/2 cup coconut milk
- 1/2 cup pineapple juice

Instructions:

1. Add all ingredients to a blender.
2. Blend until smooth.
3. Serve chilled.

Nutrition Information (per serving):

- Calories: 180
- Protein: 1g
- Carbohydrates: 40g
- Fat: 5g
- Fiber: 3g
- Sugar: 30g
- Portion Size: 1 cup

Strawberry and Basil Smoothie

Ingredients:

- 1 cup strawberries

- 5-6 basil leaves

- 1 cup Greek yogurt

- 1 tablespoon honey

Instructions:

1. Combine all ingredients in a blender.

2. Blend until smooth.

3. Serve immediately.

Nutrition Information (per serving):

- Calories: 150

- Protein: 7g

- Carbohydrates: 25g

- Fat: 3g

- Fiber: 2g

- Sugar: 20g

- Portion Size: 1.5 cups

Oatmeal Breakfast Smoothie

Ingredients:

- 1/2 cup rolled oats

- 1 banana

- 1 cup milk (dairy or plant-based)

- 1 tablespoon peanut butter

- 1 teaspoon honey

Instructions:

1. Place all ingredients in a blender.

2. Blend until smooth and creamy.

3. Pour into a glass and enjoy.

Nutrition Information (per serving):

- Calories: 300

- Protein: 9g

- Carbohydrates: 50g

- Fat: 8g

- Fiber: 6g

- Sugar: 20g

- Portion Size: 1.5 cups

CONCLUSION

In closing, this cookbook serves as a beacon of support and guidance for individuals embarking on their journey towards managing type 1 diabetes through the power of vegetarian cuisine. Throughout these pages, we've not only provided a diverse array of delicious recipes but also imparted essential knowledge on nutrition, meal planning, and the symbiotic relationship between diabetes management and a vegetarian lifestyle.

As you reflect on the culmination of this culinary adventure, remember that each recipe represents a step towards greater well-being and empowerment in managing your health. Embrace the flavors, textures, and nourishment these dishes offer, knowing that they are crafted with care to support your journey.

Beyond the kitchen, this book symbolizes a community united in the pursuit of healthier, happier lives. Whether you're a novice cook or a seasoned chef, may the recipes within these pages inspire creativity, joy, and a newfound appreciation for the incredible fusion of health and taste.

As you continue on your path, remember that you are not alone. Reach out to fellow readers, healthcare professionals, and loved ones for support, encouragement, and shared experiences. Together, we can navigate the complexities of type 1 diabetes with grace, resilience, and a hearty appetite for life.

So here's to you, to your health, and to the countless meals yet to be savored. May this cookbook be a trusted companion on your journey towards a vibrant, fulfilling life, one delicious bite at a time.